Survival Medicine:

Medicine Guide to Preparing Your First Aid Kit and Getting Completely Ready to Survive

Disclaimer: All photos used in this book, including the cover photo were made available under a Attribution-Non Commercial-Share Alike 2.0 Generic and sourced from Flickr

Table of content:

- Introduction: The Basics of Health 5
- Chapter 1: Prepping Your First Aid Survival Kit 6
  - Latex Gloves 6
  - Bandages and Field Dressing 7
  - Eye wash solution 7
  - Mild Pain Reliever 8
  - Prescription Medication 8
  - Clean Water Prep 9
  - Soap Supply 9
  - Food Prep 10
  - Clothing Prep 10
  - Basic Medical Supplies 11
  - Get a Go Bag 11
- Chapter 2: Making Use of Herbal Medicine 13
  - Herbal Nettle Leaf 13
  - Herbal Local Honey 14
  - Herbal Turmeric 14
  - Herbal Milk Thistle 15
  - Herbal Red Clover 15
  - Herbal Yarrow 16
  - Herbal Guduchi 16
  - Herbal 17
  - Herbal Anise 17
  - Herbal Chervil 18
  - Herbal Cloves 18
  - Herbal Sage 19

Chapter 3: Soothing Survival Salves 20
    Almond Lip Salve 20
    Coconut Salve 20
    Lemon Balm Salve 21
    Cat's Claw Salve 21
    Burdock Root 22
    Aloe Vera 22
    Dandelion 23
    Ashwagandha 24

Chapter 4: Aromatherapy as Survival Medicine 25
    Frankincense Oil 25
    Jasmine Oil 26
    Peppermint Oil 26
    Coriander Oil 27
    Grapefruit Oil 27
    Neroli Oil 28
    Cyprus Oil 28
    Basil Oil 29
    Bergamot Oil 29
    Fennel Oil 30

Chapter 5: Emergency Preps and Procedures 31
    How to Move the Unconscious and Injured 31
    Administering CPR 32
    Applying a Tourniquet 33
    Giving Heimlich Maneuver 34
    Treating Broken Bones and Fractures 35

Conclusion: Get Ready to Survive! 36

Introduction: The Basics of Health

As a living organism on this planet, our health tends to supersede everything else that we do. When we wake up in the morning how we feel, will directly dictate our day. If we are sluggish and groggy with a 3 day old head cold, we just aren't going to be too productive down at the office. Simply put, if we are not healthy, we are not going to be happy.

Health is intrinsically linked with everything we do. If you can keep yourself in the right physical state, you will be much better predisposed to be in the right mental state. So it is that the basics of our health are the basis of happiness itself. If you want to be healthy both mind and body in order to survive an emergency, lets get down to the basics of health!

Chapter 1: Prepping Your First Aid Survival Kit

First Aid Kits are the ultimate in survival medicine. No matter the situation, a serious injury could put you out of business pretty fast. So make sure that you have a readily accessible kit with all the staples of basic survival medicine included. In this chapter we will discuss all the best ways that you can prep your own first aid kit.

Latex Gloves

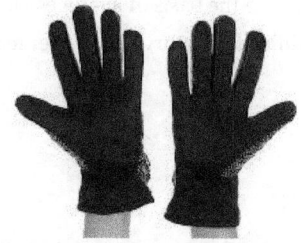

During medical emergency latex gloves could serve a wide variety of purpose. Number one they are a great way to avoid contamination if you have to deal with sick members of your household or any other known for of contagion. These gloves are also ideal for cleaning as well so that your hands can remain free from dangerous cleaning chemicals.

Another good time to use latex gloves would be in the preparation of medicine, since you don't want to inadvertently absorb medication through your skin. Latex glove are the strongest and most versatile gloves to use for this purpose. These gloves can be found at just about any department store so feel free to stock up on a few pairs.

Bandages and Field Dressing

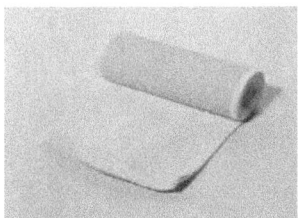

We all get banged up from to time to time. We could stumble and fall, we could get burned, and we can break bones. It is a dangerous world and when you are in a true survival situation these injuries need to be addressed on the spot. Having that said having fresh bandages and some sort of immediate dressing you can immediately put to use is of tremendous importance.

Eye wash solution

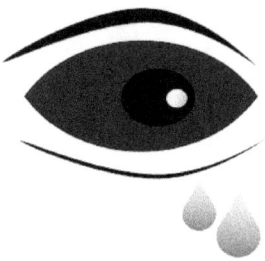

Our eyes are the window to the soul and if those windows become foggy we are not going to be able to function as well as we should in our time of need. Your eyes could become clouded with debris, infected, or otherwise compromised. The best way to counteract this is to have a strong saline solution that you can spritz right into your eyes when needed. A simple squeeze or spray bottle applied directly to the bottom eye lid should do the trick just fine.

Mild Pain Reliever

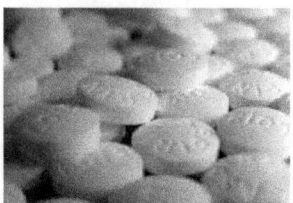

It's very important to pack a mild pain reliever in your first aid kit and it shouldn't be neglected. Anything from aspirin to Tylenol should be included for any minor aches and pains that might be experienced. This mild kind of mild pain reliever is good at reducing fever and treating headaches, as well as helping to counteract back aches, ankle sprains and a whole host of other issues. So yes, make sure you pack some of this great pain relief in your First Aid Survival Kit.

Prescription Medication

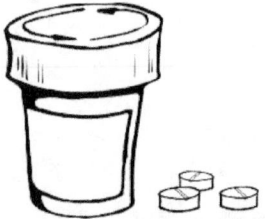

It should go without saying that it would be of some great use for you pack your prescription medication with your First Aid Kit. In a time of crisis you may not be able to go to the local pharmacy to get that prescription filled at the last minute, so you should make sure that you have a proper supply on hand at all times. Many said stories have transpired regarding those that due not prepare for this contingence, so make sure that you are not one of them.

Clean Water Prep

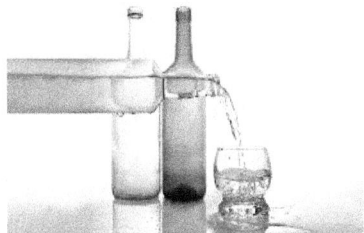

Having a clean supply of drinking water is one of the first things that anyone should strive for when they are prepping their survival first aid kit. And if you can't stock up on clean water, then you should at least pack the rudiments of how you can *create your own clean water*. This means that you should pack chlorine tablets, water filters, and perhaps something to boil the H2O in, just to make sure that your water is appropriately prepped for consumption.

Soap Supply

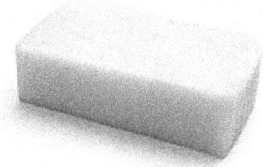

Packing soap in your First Aid Survival Kit isn't so much for good hygiene and making yourself presentable as it is for making sure that injuries don't get worse. Don't get me wrong, being clean is good, but being able to clean out your wounds is even better. And for any injury or infection that you might have to deal with in the aftermath of an emergency you will need to make sure that the area of injury is kept as clean as possible.

Food Prep

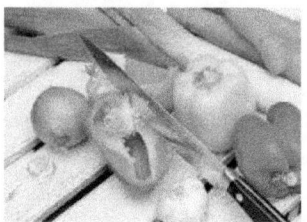

While you shouldn't cram a four course meal in your First Aid Survival Kit, it would be a good idea to place some very basic staples inside it. Your First Aid Survival Kit should contain such basic necessities as flour, salt, sugar, bullion cubes, and dry pasta. It's not much, but these simple morsels could be of great use if you are caught up in a prolonged crisis in which getting regular groceries proves to be a difficult proposition.

Clothing Prep

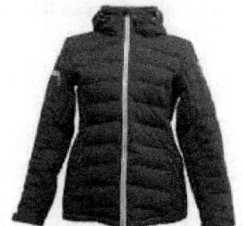

Any good First Aid Survival Kit should have appropriate clothing supplies in packed away within them. This means that your kit should have room for at least one pair of clean clothing to change into. This is of use in case all of your other clothes become inaccessible or are otherwise compromised. It is also a good idea to pack some heavier winter type clothing in case you find yourself in colder climes for an extended period.

Basic Medical Supplies

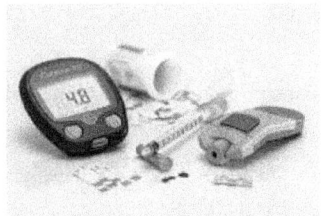

Your First Aid Survival Kit should have basic supplies such as ice packs, hydrogen peroxide, extra bandages, adhesive tape, scissors, tweezers, and thread. The latter of which are of extreme import since they can be used to sew up stitches if need be. Yes, if you find yourself badly injured you may need to take some drastic measures such as sewing up your own stitches, so be sure to bring adequate medical supplies to do so.

Get a Go Bag

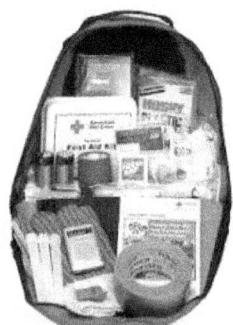

The "Go Bag" is basically a bag of items that you would grab if you had to hit the road in the hurry and is provided here as an auxiliary resource to your First Aid Survival Kit.

You should actually prep a go bag for every member of your household and identity each person's bag with either an ID tag or by—at the very least—writing their name on the outside of the bag in magic marker.

This bag should contain a good flashlight, a battery operated radio, surgical mask, small knife, bottle of water, extra shoes, socks, underwear, prescription meds, toothpaste and brush, and an extra pack of batteries. These are all great preps to help you survive the storm—whatever that storm may be.

Chapter 2: Making Use of Herbal Medicine

Antibiotics are beneficial for a wide variety of ailments and this couldn't be more than in an emergency situation. So here in this chapter we have listed for you some of the best herbal antibiotics that you could ever come by. Take note of all of their benefits and how they could be of use to you.

Herbal Nettle Leaf

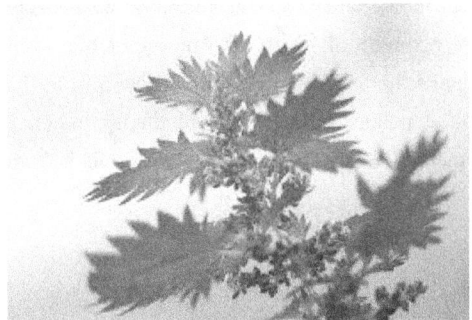

If you are facing a problem with inflammation, the healing powers of the Stinging Nettle leaf may be just what you are looking for. The Stinging Nettle provides a natural kind of antibiotic support that you can't find in very many other places. The antihistamine power of Nettle leaves can forego a running nose and eliminate fever all together. This leaf is known for its ability to reduce fevers and even get rid of the aches and pains of a toothache! If you are feeling down in the dumps, give this leaf a try.

Herbal Local Honey

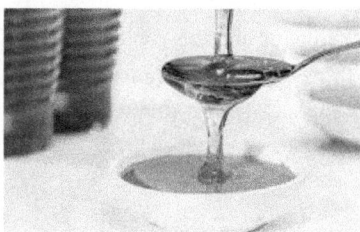

Many are not aware of it but local honey is a powerful antibiotic able to kill bacteria and reduce the affects of common allergies. The power of this local honey comes from the bees that make them. These bees ingest pollen from the environment and then by the time this pollen is transformed by them into honey it contains powerful antibiotic elements that will help shield whoever its it from regional illness. It's just that easy!

Herbal Turmeric

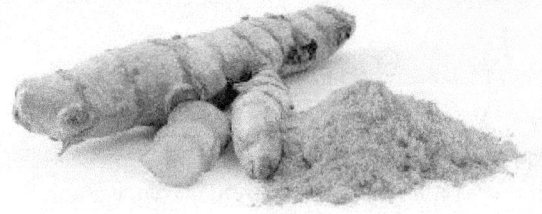

Turmeric is a great ingredient in many spicy dishes, but it that same hard biting Turmeric also serves a great purpose as an antibiotic. Turmeric has been known to reduce fevers and even prevent the onset of cold and flu viruses. A powerful ingredient called "curccumin" is the usually sighted ingredient that is capable of this feat. And the more curccumin your Turmeric has in store, the better off you will most certainly be!

Herbal Milk Thistle

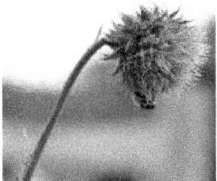

This herb is another great item to pack in your medicine chest. With its ability to reduce inflammation, this herb has been known to have some rather amazing results. Milk thistle serves to boost liver function and in some instances has even been seen to reverse the effects of cirrhosis. If you have any inflammation whatsoever, simply apply some Milk Thistle directly to the area afflicted and you will see results.

Herbal Red Clover

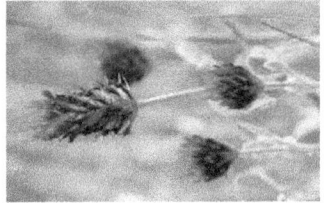

Red Clover is a powerful herbal antibiotic that can greatly boost the immune system. This herb has even been known to increase the red blood cell count in those that use it. Interestingly enough, Red Clover is also a natural anticoagulant and can loosen up blood clots in rather rapid fashion. This in turn provides a general boost in health no matter what you may be facing.

Herbal Yarrow

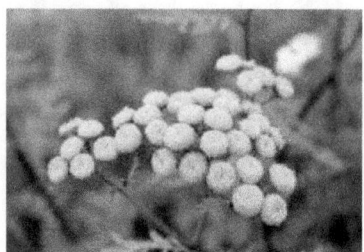

Yarrow is an herb that has been used for centuries; and with good reason. This herb can get to work on inflammation and congestion in the human body, almost immediately. This herbal antibiotic also works well against injuries, and as soon as it is applied to a injured site, it gets to work cleansing the injury and promoting the formation for blood platelets for a quick and effective healing.

Herbal Guduchi

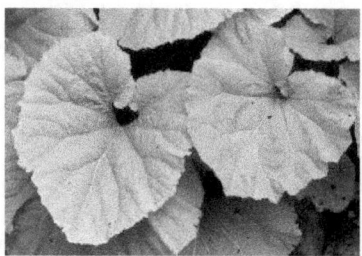

This herb is a great antibiotic fighter and its best work is done to reduce inflammation and boost the immune system. Just apply a small amount of this herbal antibiotic to the skin and you will be able to enhance your body's ability to stand up to and survive all manner of airborne illnesses. Give this herbal Guduchi Antibiotic a try!

Herbal

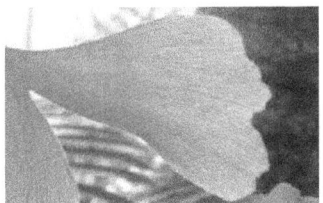

Ginkgo is a powerful and useful allergy fighter and works to reduce inflammation. This herb is also great when it comes to improving the flow of oxygen to the brain. It is for this reason that so many take Ginkgo to boost their memory and concentration. So if you are feeling at all slow and sluggish in the morning—or any other time for that matter—a good dose of Ginkgo tea could really do you some good! This tea can be made through either boiling powdered Ginkgo or raw Ginkgo leaves.

Herbal Anise

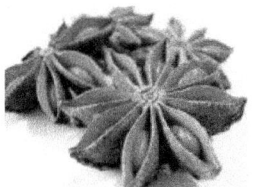

This herb works out just great as an herbal antibiotic, killing most bacteria right on the spot. This herbal antibiotic also works on the urinary system, helping to clear up any incontinence that someone may be facing, and putting the whole body into a kind of detox, almost immediately. One of the best ways to administer this healing herb is to boil it into a nice and tasty tea. So drink up folks because this Herbal Anise is on me!

Herbal Chervil

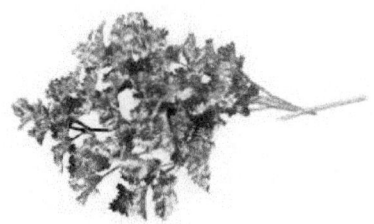

Chervil has a real proven ability when it comes to killing bacteria, getting rid of headaches and calming upset stomachs. It is the latter from which many a camper has benefited. It is common practice for many survivalists to simply pop a leaf of chervil in their mouth and chew in order to relieve their upset stomach. I have tried this myself and can say that it really does wonders.

Herbal Cloves

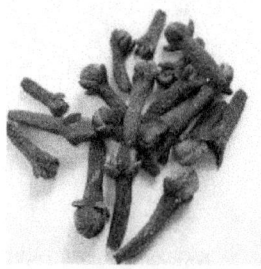

In a similar fashion to chervil, cloves have been placed directly into the mouth of many dental patients in order to kill bacteria and curb inflammatory agents. This herb also works as a mild form of pain reliever and can be used to successfully numb up a bad toothache if needed.

Herbal Sage

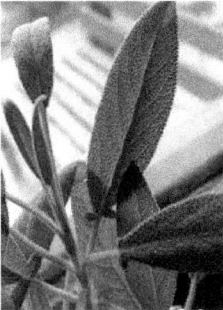

This medicinal herb takes survival medicine to a whole new live in the way that it can successfully reduce all manner of pain and kill bacterial infections on the spot. If you have fallen and sustained an injury, just a very small application of this healing herb will work to alleviate any pain that you may feel. Another great benefit of herbal sage is its ability to treat asthma. I have suffered with asthma most of my life myself, and applications of this herb have helped to improve my own breathing considerably when I have tried it.

Chapter 3: Soothing Survival Salves

Here are a few healing salves that will help you survive just about anything that comes your way!

Almond Lip Salve

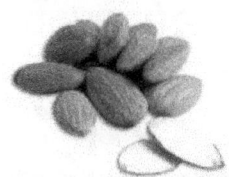

This healing salve is a natural way to cure dry lips. If you have repeatedly dry and cracking lips you can greatly benefit by even the smallest of applications of this herbal lip balm. This lip balm is almost odorless and has just a slightly sweet taste that will not interfere with eating or anything else you do throughout the course of a day.

Coconut Salve

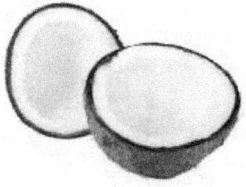

Coconut salves are always classy and soothing. This salve is no exception. Made out of concentrated coconut oil, just a little dab will do you! Place this coconut salve on your lips, feet, arms, or any other part of your being that could use just a little bit of soothing!

Lemon Balm Salve

Lemon Balm is perhaps one of the most popular salves that you could ever use. These salves are great for chapped lips and even better for rough hands. You can also use this salve as an herbal antibiotic since lemon naturally kills all germs and bacteria on contact. Lemon balm salve is also great for the face and even small applications of it can help can clear up complexions and even treat wrinkling of the skin.

Cat's Claw Salve

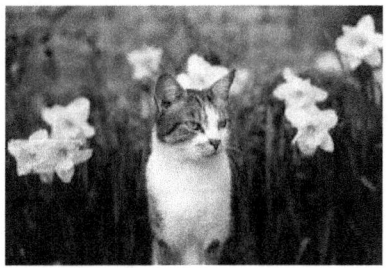

This healing salve is a great immune booster and can even help promote the production of white blood cells when regularly applied to the skin. Simply put; external viruses, bacteria, and other germs don't stand a chance when cat's claw is applied!

Burdock Root

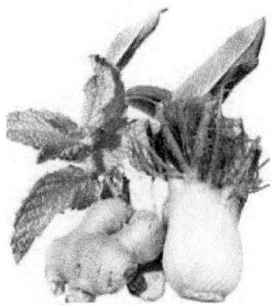

If you are suffering from arthritis, the inflammation fighting power of a little Burdock Root could be just what the doctor ordered for you. Just a brief application of this healing salve and your arthritis will be long behind you. Be sure to pack this herbal healing salve in your bag as part of your survival medicine arsenal.

Aloe Vera

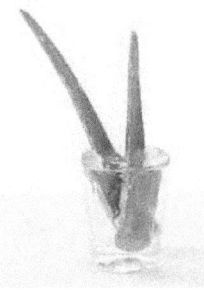

Burns have met their match with Aloe Vera. This healing salve sooths even as it protects. As soon as you apply Aloe Vera to a burn on the skin you will feel the soothing relief that this herb can provide. Burns by their nature—as well as damaging tissue structure—take all of the moisture out of the injury.

But an application of Aloe Vera will put that moisture back in. So don't hesitate to bring yourself some Aloe Vera folks! The best way to pack it is in a tube, but *if you can hack it*, you can make some of your own. All you have to do is take the Aloe Vera leaf, split it open and then scoop the gel out. Either way you will have a powerful and soothing herbal healing salve on your hands.

Dandelion

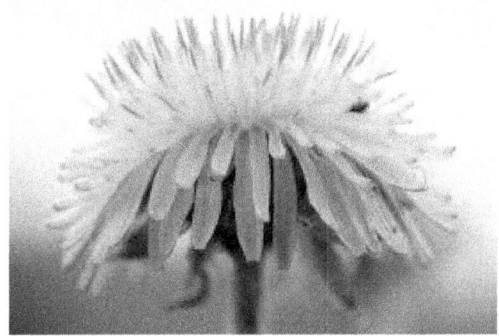

Dandelions are quite prolific, you see than sprouting up in yards, parking lots and businesses all across the country. The bane of lawnmowers and weed whackers everywhere—these little yellow guys really do get around.

And this healing salve once applied can do wonders for everything from allergies to immune system protection. Improving the production of platelets in the blood, this healing salve has been shown to even improve the lives of cancer patients. So this is definitely a survival medicine tat could be of some great use for you.

Ashwagandha

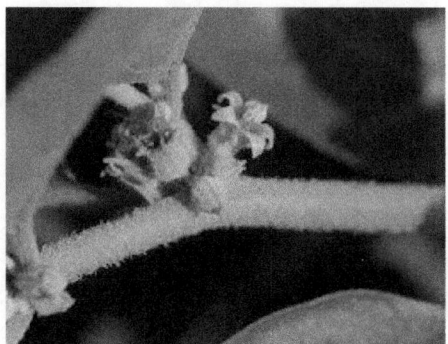

This healing salve has been with us for quite some time, and known as an "adaptogen" it can work to adapt to just about any situation that is thrown at it. Ashwagandha can help with everything from inflammation, to boosting immune health, to healing injuries from cuts, scrapes, and burns. All of this makes for some great soothing survival salves!

Chapter 4: Aromatherapy as Survival Medicine

Aromatherapy is an ancient practice with powerful results for modern survival medicine. Just take a look at the following examples and how they can greatly enrich your life—no matter the situation.

Frankincense Oil

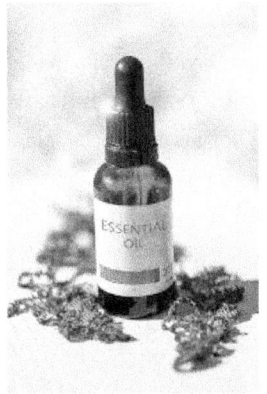

Frankincense has a long history of use. It was prized in ancient times both for its alluring aroma and for its healing properties. Just rub this essential oil into the skin and the healing properties of this herb will work to holistically treat your entire body. It boosts the immune system and cleanses at the same time.

In order to administer Frankincense Oil, either breathe in the aroma from a fresh bottle of essential oil or place a few drops in an incense burner and let the aroma fill the entire room, so that you can benefit from the treatment gradually as you go about your day.

Jasmine Oil

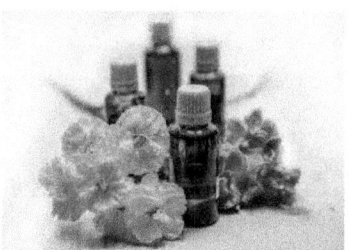

Jasmine has quite a lovely aroma and most that have breathed it in will agree to how refreshing it can be. And when you concentrate the oil of jasmine down to its most powerful form for aroma therapy the effects can be downright life changing. This essential oil has been known to boost memory and overall mental focus for those that use it. Just breathe in a few drops of this stuff and you will know the true meaning of aromatherapy for survival medicine.

Peppermint Oil

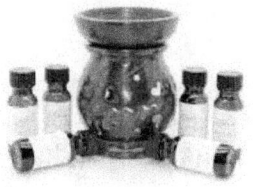

This refreshing blast of peppermint will help to calm your nerves and maybe even boost your metabolism! Peppermint is also known to open up the breathing passages so if you are having any trouble with congestion of shortness of breath, you may want to seriously give peppermint a try. As an asthma sufferer myself I can attest to the healing power of peppermint. Just a few whiffs of this stuff and I am all better. So be sure to keep some of this wondrous healing herb on hand for your own survival medicine.

Coriander Oil

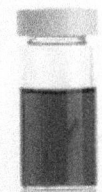

I was first exposed to coriander oil as something to cook with. But little did I know that coriander oil is also great for aromatherapy. Just by breathing in the aroma of this oil you will be able to greatly increase the blood supply of your cardiovascular system. This extra burst of blood flow will actually help your body to relax considerably. So if you feel like may need a break, just breathe in some coriander oil.

Grapefruit Oil

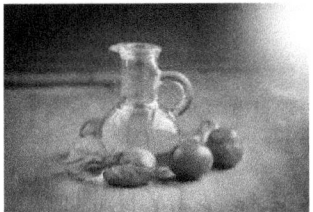

The powerful aromatherapy provided by grapefruit oil can work to really get you going in the morning! This essential oil when breathed in directly will allow for your body to get that extra boost it needs to get through the day. Regular regimens of breathing in this oil could also greatly improve your mental clarity and recall of events. So yes, I would advise, if you need survival medicine, then you need to give some grapefruit oil a try!

Neroli Oil

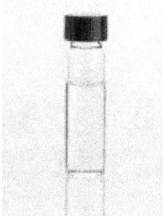

The effect of this essential oil when breathed into the body through a regular routine of aromatherapy is almost immediate. As soon as you breathe it in you will begin to feel your heart beat just a little bit slower. And after your treatment progresses your whole body will soon be relaxed! Neroli oil is highly recommended!

Cyprus Oil

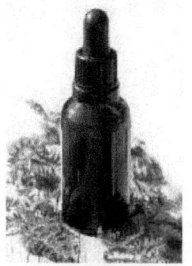

You may have noticed the scent of cypress in many cars you have been driven in since Cyprus is the number one scent in car air fresheners. You may have had the privilege of sitting under a tree shaped car air freshener and breathed in that tree-like scent. Well this essential oil is also quite effective as a form of aromatic treatment for a wide range of illnesses and discomforts.

Most notably this aromatic oil is great for giving those who breathe it in a refreshing calm and an increase in overall energy. So if you need a bit of a boost at any time during yo9ur day you should just take some time to stop and smell the Cyprus!

Basil Oil

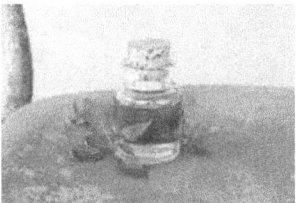

Basil is a great ingredient in many cuisines, but it is also a valuable aromatic agent in its own right. Basil oil is quite often used to boost the immune system, aid concentration, and relax the senses. Believe me—just put a few drops of basil oil in your incense burner and you will be feeling better in no time.

Bergamot Oil

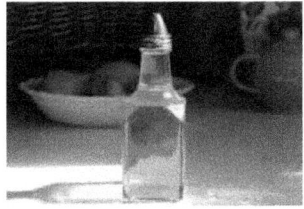

This essential oil is great for relieving cramps. People don't realize it, but muscle cramps and spasms are not just a minor inconvenience they can actually be life threatening.

And if you are in an emergency situation to where you need to walk and run away from something, a cramped up leg is going to get you in a lot of trouble real quick.

Well then—if you need to straighten up a badly cramped leg, a good dose of bergamot oil can do the trick for you. Just breathe in the aroma direct from the bottle or put a couple of drops in your incense burner and you will be in good shape in no time.

Fennel Oil

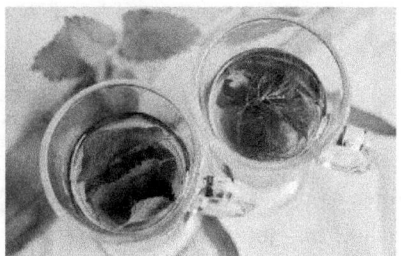

This oil works to improve the immune system and overall metabolic function of the body. If you are in a crisis situation or prolonged emergency in which regular health treatment may not be available, being able to administer aromatherapy with this oil could be crucial. In order to administer your own fennel oil just breathe the aroma direct or add it to an incense burner or similar distribution device.

Chapter 5: Emergency Preps and Procedures

During a medical emergency you have precious few minutes to figure what to do. And last minute crash courses in brain surgery aren't going to be too beneficial. So here it is in this chapter, a full listing of emergency preps and procedures that you just might find useful in the midst of a perilous situation.

How to Move the Unconscious and Injured

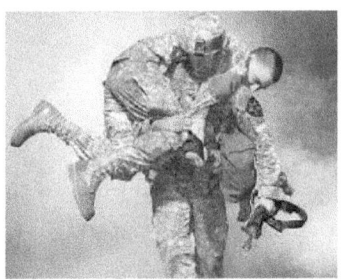

If someone you are with becomes seriously hurt you may need to assist them by moving them from location to location. Having that said, this means that you need to know the *proper way* to move them. If there are signs of a back injury for example, you need to make sure that the patient is rendered immobile in order to prevent any further injury to the back and neck. If you have someone to help you lift this person, that's great, but if you are by yourself you may just have to improvise.

One easy way to move someone would be to use a large article of clothing such as a bed sheet, or large coat to drag the individual. This is done by wrapping the clothing securely around the person's legs. You can then pull your ailing comrade to safety, it may not be the prettiest or most sophisticated way to render aid, but when all else fails, it will get the job done.

Administering CPR

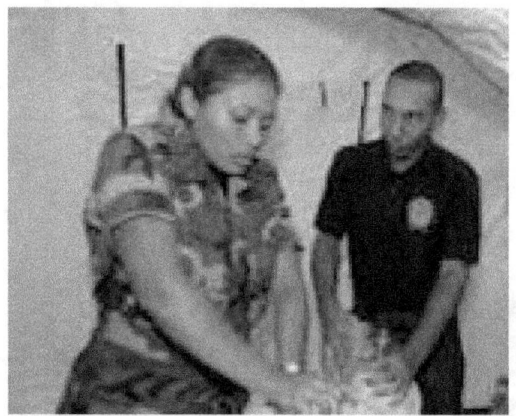

Standing for "cardiopulmonary resuscitation", the technique called CPR is used to apply manual pressure to a heart that has stopped beating. In order to apply CPR, make sure the patient is on their back, on a flat surface. Now kneel beside the patient, positioning in line with their chest. Now place your index finger at the bottom notch of the person's ribs.

Position your hand's heel above this notch. Now place the palm of your hand on top of the other positioned above the notch. Now you can begin your chest compressions. Use a compression rate of 80 to 100 per minute, and stop every 15 to breathe 2 breaths into the person's lungs in between compressions. This emergency prep could be invaluable during a crisis.

Applying a Tourniquet

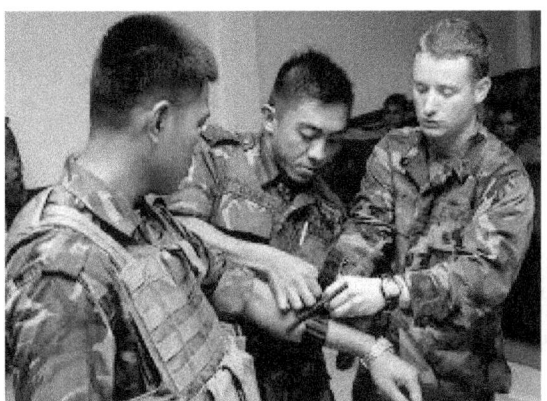

It's a gruesome reality, but if someone is injured severely enough, they can bleed to death. In order to prevent a tragedy like this, you need to know how to apply a tourniquet. Tourniquet's can be self applied or applied to others, and simply consist of a material being wrapped around a limb in order to apply pressure and stem the flow of bleeding.

You can make a simple tourniquet simply by ripping a strip of cloth off of your shirt and tying it tightly around the affected area. Make sure the material is at least an inch and a half wide to make sure that it doesn't break and will remain stable. Keep this tourniquet on until you can stabilize the patient.

Giving Heimlich Maneuver

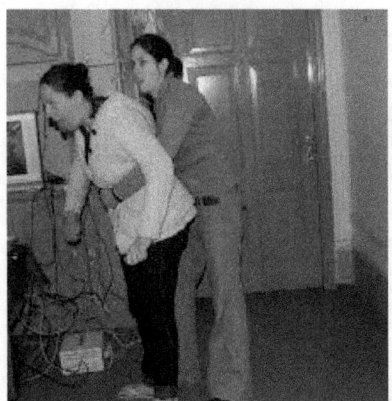

If you see someone with a look of clear distress, with their face contorted in fear, unable to speak, unable to even breathe, and they are pointing to their throat, you can be sure that they are choking. In such a desperate situation the Heimlich maneuver is just what the survival doctor ordered. In order to properly administer this life saving maneuver, you need to stand directly behind the choking victim and place your arms around their stomach as if you are giving them a hug.

Now ball your hand into a fist and grab the outside of this fist with your other hand. Now with your elbows pointed out behind you begin energetically thrusting that fist up into the person's stomach causing the wind to shoot up through their diaphragm. This will eventually cause whatever is obstructing their windpipe to shoot out of their mouth. This bit of survival medicine really could save someone's life.

Treating Broken Bones and Fractures

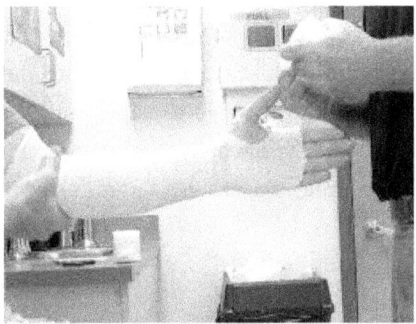

Broken bones and fractures can happen to anyone, so in order to make your survival medicine effective, you need to be able to know how to treat a common contingency such as this. If you or someone else in your company breaks or fractures a bone, the first thing that needs to be done is to stabilize the injury so that no further damage occurs.

This means putting arms in slings and legs in casts where necessary. Immobilize these injured body parts in the exact position you found them in, don't attempt to re-position the broken bones as this could cause further harm. So yes, be prepared to mobilize the individuals broken or fractured bones in the position in which you found them, this will help prevent further injury until they can receive further treatment.

Conclusion: Get Ready to Survive!

Preparing for the unpredictable is not an oxymoron it is simply being proactive in a troubled world. And in any crisis situation our health should be of number one concern to us. That was my purpose in writing this book to give the reader an inside look at just what kind of emergency medicines and procedures so that they may be ready. And readiness is indeed a good thing. So take these words to heart and go ahead and get ready to survive!

www.ingramcontent.com/pod-product-compliance
Lightning Source LLC
Chambersburg PA
CBHW050251230526
45470CB00005B/2215